Who Needs Hair...

The FLIP Side of Chemotherapy

by

Sallie Astor Burdine

with illustrations by
Rebecca Kieler

SABA Books
Bluewater Bay, Florida

Published by:
SABA BOOKS
P.O. Box 5265
Bluewater Bay, Florida 32578

This information is for general health information only and is not intended to be a substitute for professional medical advice, diagnosis or treatment. All specific medical questions should be presented to your own health care provider.

The purpose of this manual is to educate and entertain. The author and Saba Books shall have neither liability nor responsibility to any person or entity with respect to any loss or damage caused, or alleged to be caused, directly or indirectly by the information contained in this book. If you do not wish to be bound by the above, you may return this book to the publisher for a full refund.

ISBN: 0-9705464-8-3
Library of Congress Catalog Card Number: 2001116884
Cover, Book Design and Production by Pearl & Associates, Inc.
Illustrations by Rebecca Kieler
Back cover photograph by Elizabeth Watson
Printed and Manufactured in the United States of America

Who Needs Hair...

What others are saying...

"Good medicine for those of us whose lives are changed by cancer, *Who Needs Hair...the Flip side of Chemotherapy*, brings laughter and even, joy, to what is otherwise a sad time."

—Dr. Joe Pulliam, M.D.

llie Burdine offers a good strong dose of positive energy what can be a vastly negative situation."

—Desiree Lyon, Board Member,
MD Anderson Cancer Center

"This much-needed book amazingly integrates smiles with the tears and fears of the cancer experience."

—Alinda C. Sledge, MSW, ACSW, LCSW,
Professor of Social Work

"*Who Needs Hair...the Flip side of Chemotherapy* successfully reaffirms what most cancer patients will soon discover: the trivial becomes all the more trivial and the important becomes all the more important."

—Anthony Herrera, Actor, Producer,
Writer, Cancer Survivor

"For the hundreds of thousands of women who will be diagnosed with cancer this year and for the millions who still live with cancer...this book gives hope and a positive view of their plight in life."

—Tom Redmond, Board Member,
National Prostate Cancer Coalition

It has been said that cancer patients are among the bravest people in the world. This doesn't mean they are not afraid – just that they possess vast amounts of courage.

To all of you, I dedicate this book.

And especially to the memory of
Fidelia Alexander,
Johnny Yurkow,
and Ken Berk
Three PROS at looking for the FLIP side

And for Jasmine, who is strong and well
from Becky, with love

Note to the Reader

If you have received this book as a gift, it is my hope that you regard

it as a means to uplift you. As you may or may not have figured out

by now, in your journey through cancer, the people around you

respond to your crisis in various and sundry ways. Some may fall to

pieces, some may rally around you with love and support and, for

whatever reason, some may not respond at all. One thing you can be

sure of, though, is that the person who gave you this book—simply

hoped to make you smile.

Contents

Acknowledgments

With Much Gratitude

To my children, Matt, Ben and Alden

You have always amazed me, but never so profoundly as the way you have handled my cancer. With rare wisdom and understanding, you have accepted the strange reality that while cancer may threaten your mother's life, it has also enriched ALL of our lives – by deepening our love for one another and by offering a new appreciation for the beauty of everyday life. So thank you with all my heart. You have not only shared me with the huge and often scary world of cancer, but you have allowed me time and quiet to share myself with others whose walk will follow mine.

To my husband, Hank

You have filled in the missing pieces of the puzzle of my life and just when I thought all was complete, another void or complexity presented itself in the form of cancer. But again, you remind me that life is not a destination, but a journey. And, oh, my love, I thank you for always accompanying me on my journeys, no matter how difficult -- YOU are there for me. This book would not exist had it not been for your love and support, nor would most things I value in my life. I love you eternally.

To my truest soul sisters, Mary Ellen Hammett, Sherry Smythe, Emily Crowley, Judy Jernigan, Alinda Sledge, Carla Barnes and Audrey Gluschke,

I can never thank you enough for utterly stopping your lives and investing your time and money into never letting me face one moment of the cancer world alone. You arrived in Houston with blenders, wigs, funny movies, etc. and turned my nightmare into an adventure. With your usual love, strength and humor, you gave me all I ever needed to stay focused on the Flip side, which kept me hanging in there with this book AND my recovery.

To my parents, Fred and Jane Astor, *for showering me with optimism from the day I was born.*
To my brother, Rick Astor, *for his strength, support, love and encouragement.*
To my precious niece, Kristin Joseph, *my sunshine who shined ever so brightly while living with me during chemo.*

To Tom and Cher Redmond, *for insisting I go to MD Anderson Cancer Center and then accompanying me through all the many facets.*

To Dick and Desiree Howe, *for adopting me into their mighty network of healing – which God manifests through their faith and the brilliance of MD Anderson Cancer Center.*

To Dr. Nuhad Ibrahim, M.D., *my trusted oncologist, my realistic yet optimistic physician – who exudes the rare combination of brilliance with just the right amount of compassion, patience and humor.*

To Becky Kieler, esteemed artist, *for her expertise and willingness to draw my sometimes-ridiculous visions with no expectations, but with simple joy.*

To Carol Jolley, *my dear new friend and on-call consultant for this project*

To Sandy Pearlman, my editor *for her keen eye and expertise*

To Ronald T. Smith, President of Bookworld, *for not being too busy or too important to take my call -- only to tell me the brutal truth… and then giving me the chance of a lifetime.*

And last but not least, ***to Chris Pearl, of Pearl Design and Associates,*** *master cover and lay-out designer, publisher consultant and advisor – a HUGE thank you for gently, yet firmly taking the reins and leading this book to completion.*

Introduction

WHO NEEDS HAIR? I DO! I need it because my status as a chemo patient has rendered me bald. I need it because my sickly white scalp clashes with what I thought to be my healthy face. I need it because my head gets cold at night. And, darn it, I need my hair because I've never been without it!

I have lived forty-six years with a head full of hair, along with two ears, two eyes, one nose and a mouth. Hair is normal. It's expected. It's part of the human anatomy, for goodness sake. And now mine is gone. All gone — except for a yellow tuft of loyal renegades who refuse to fall out. I guess it's the razor for them — unless I want to try the electrocuted baby-chick look.

Introduction

So, how did I get this way? How did you? Unfortunately, nobody knows for sure why you and I got to be the unlucky recipients of this widespread epidemic we call cancer.

The point is, I don't ask "why me?" anymore. The real question is, *"Why not me?"* As a patient at M.D. Anderson Cancer Center, where they see over 7000 patients a week, I can tell you firsthand that cancer knows no boundaries. Old and young, rich and poor, all races, all religions. Going to a checkup or to treatment at M.D. Anderson is like attending a conference at the World Trade Center.

Of all the special interest groups in the world, I would think we cancer patients have the largest numbers. Well, at least our dilemma is socially accepted, well funded and continues to be in the limelight.

QUOTE

You are not alone
The National Cancer Institute estimates that approximately 8.4 million Americans alive today have a history of cancer. Some of these individuals can be considered cured, while others still have evidence of cancer and may be undergoing treatment.

—2000 Cancer Facts & Figures AMC

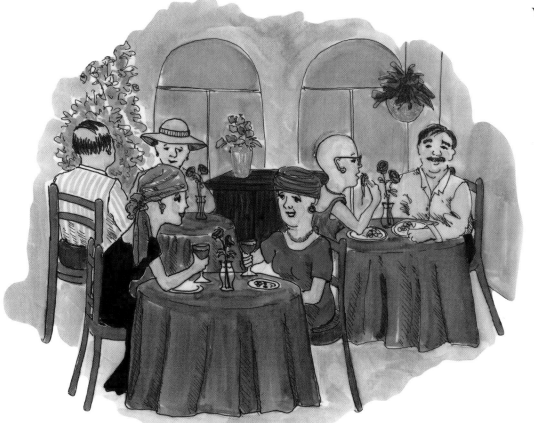

"My dear daughter, didn't you know?
These days, you're not in style if you don't have cancer.

Introduction

Nevertheless, getting back to needing hair, I do need my hair, but I especially need to live a healthy and, hopefully, long life. Cancer seriously threatens this, and believe me, I would do just about anything to get rid of it once and for all.

This hostile invader has zapped my body, scared my soul and attempted to destroy my life. It is possibly the most relentless and terrifying of all terrorists, and never before have tears and fears overcome me with such vigilance.

Having said that, though — as I sit here with my eyebrows and eyelashes falling out, I figure I can simply drown in all this misery or I can keep swimming and somehow keep my hairless head above water. Thus, this is a book about the brighter side, the sunny side,

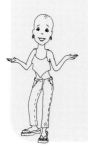

QUOTE

*"Pain is inevitable,
misery is optional"*

—anonymous

the flip side of cancer. Can this be true? Is there such a side to a

plight so dark and terrifying?

I know there is because I found it, and in so doing, I can now

endure my cancer and its required chemotherapy a little bit better. I

still have to live with it day by day, but it's more tolerable now, as I

focus on the serious and not-so-serious blessings I have discovered

within my curse.

None of us will escape agony and tragedy in our individual lives, and

granted, some experiences are so painful one would not even

attempt to find good in such misfortune. Yet, with the majority of

calamity(s), if we look hard enough, there is usually a fleck of gold

buried somewhere in our suffering.

Introduction

It will take courage to search for it, but in so doing, we may find that this golden light can warm and brighten even the coldest, most dismal dilemma we face. This is not to minimize the pain, or desensitize others to our anguish, but to help us find something, *anything,* to smile about, to muse about in the midst of our discomfort.

We've all heard a zillion times about the power of positive thinking. Attitude is everything! As a man thinketh, so shall he be! It's how we respond that's important. I know, it's nauseating enough to just go through chemotherapy without all that, so I'll stop. But I do believe that humor, gratitude and faith can go a long way toward making the worst of days a little bit — and sometimes a lot — better.

QUOTE

Happy is the man and happy he alone,
He who is secure within can say:
"Tomorrow doesn't matter, for I have lived today."

—Horace

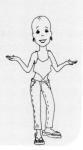

QUOTE

A cheerful heart is truly good medicine

—Proverbs 17:22

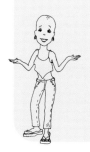

It is with this in mind that I beseech you, as one cancer patient to another, to look for what I call the flip side. Search for that little ray of sunshine and, just maybe, not all of your days will be as dark and difficult.

I still have days when the positive and funny parts of being bald cannot outweigh the negative parts of cancer. These are the days when I accept my fear and misery without a fight. But on the other days, a little humor, along with a swift kick in the rear, goes a long way toward keeping my bare head above water.

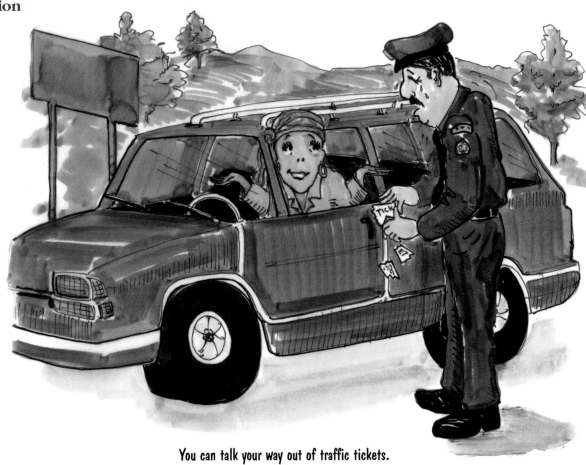

You can talk your way out of traffic tickets.

In the Beginning

As I look back to the days and weeks following my diagnosis of cancer, I recall family and friends scurrying around me, frantically searching for a fix, a cure, if you will, to save me from a death sentence. Medical personnel were also a constant presence, drifting in and out of my hospital room — without the panic and urgency of my loved ones but with a certain consistency to hit the nail on its head.

Where did the malignancy begin? How far and to where had it metastasized? These were the questions being asked

In the Beginning

and the purpose of the many tests I would endure.

Somehow, I remember feeling as if I wasn't really there.

Everyone was talking about me or at least my body parts —

breasts, lymph nodes, organs, bones, etc. — as they ruled

in and out where the cancer was and wasn't.

Within days, I was sent home from the hospital to recover

from my biopsy, which included the removal of thirty-two

malignant lymph nodes. I remember floating about as the

phone rang constantly and well-meaning friends and family

began to quarrel over which hospital, which oncologist,

whether or not I should have a mastectomy, etc.

QUOTE

There are as many nights as days, and the one is just as long as the other in the year's course. Even a happy life cannot be without a measure of darkness, and the word "happiness" would lose its meaning if it were not balanced by sadness. It is far better to take things as they come along with patience and equanimity.

—Carl Gustav Jung

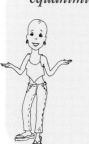

My state of mind was amazingly peaceful. A new adventure was unfolding before me, and in some strange way, I looked forward to it. It wasn't long, though, before the adventure faded into a long, slow, bad dream. My Stage Four advanced breast cancer had metastasized into my bones, and I was placed on an aggressive eight-month trial study of chemotherapy. A mastectomy and possible bone marrow transplant were left up in the air until we saw how my body would respond to the treatment.

In the Beginning

I prepared myself to face the ravages of chemotherapy by reading and by interviewing other cancer victims. However, nothing can prepare one to face what I was about to face. One must experience chemotherapy firsthand to know its harsh reality.

Within days of my first round of treatment, my hair began to fall out in handfuls. As expected, I fell into bed exhausted, bald and scared. *How was I to go on living?* I couldn't just stop my life while I waited to get well or to die. I thought I could possibly beat this thing, and if not, I was sure I could hang on for many years fighting it. *But how would I live in the meantime?*

My entire being seemed to change overnight. I was no longer the blonde, athletic, zestful, happy-go-lucky girl I once was. My past was over, my future looked grim and my present seemed futile. I don't remember wanting to die, but I do remember not wanting to wake up and face each new day. I became so miserable that I was forced to live life "moment by moment" instead of "one day at a time." This is when I began to live again.

Gradually, but beautifully, like a thousand dazzling lights slowly dancing toward me, I began to see that life does go on for cancer patients, *especially* for cancer patients.

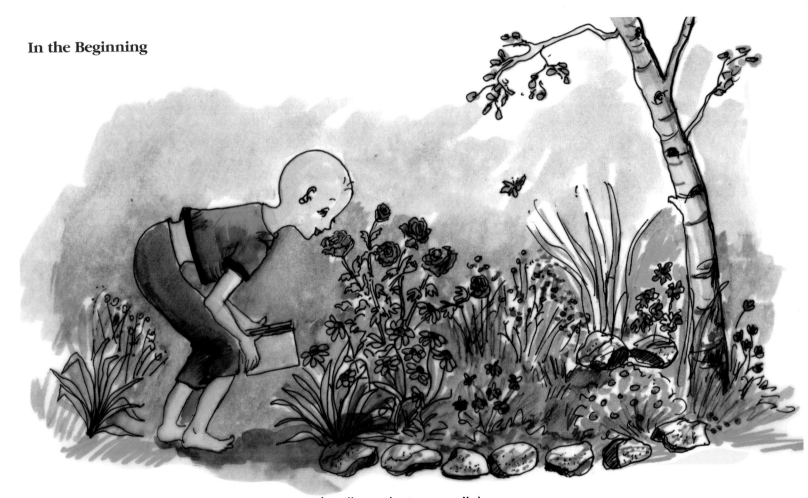

You will now take time to smell those roses.

QUOTE

One doesn't discover new lands without consenting to lose sight of the shore for a very long time.

—Andre Gide

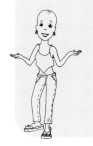

This revelation surprised me and filled me with a sense of relief the likes of which I've never felt before. It was as if a big "WHEW!" blew through my mind and emotions. I had felt the terrifying winds of change upon my diagnosis — and though the wind was still blowing, it was no longer howling.

When I got up each morning, I began the day by putting on makeup and getting dressed. I learned how to put on eyeliner and eyebrow pencil to hide my lack of eyelashes and eyebrows. I played with scarves and turbans until I found a new, dramatic "gypsy" look that gave me the confidence to go out in public again.

In the Beginning

One day I accepted an invitation to lunch. Another day I
began to take daily walks. Before I knew it, I was back to my
old self — except for one major difference. I took nothing for
granted — not a star, not a song, not a smile — nothing. Life
would never be the same for me. I could grieve or I could
celebrate. The choice was mine.

My message is this: If you are newly diagnosed with or even a
veteran of cancer, you can still go on living. Your life may be
different, but I promise you — if you are willing to try —

blessings of your own will surface as you face each new day

with a determination to live life fully and, most importantly,

with joy.

QUOTE

*It has been said that there is
no such thing as a problem
that doesn't have a gift in it.*

—Tim Hansel, *You Gotta Keep Dancin'*

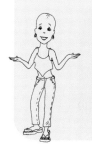

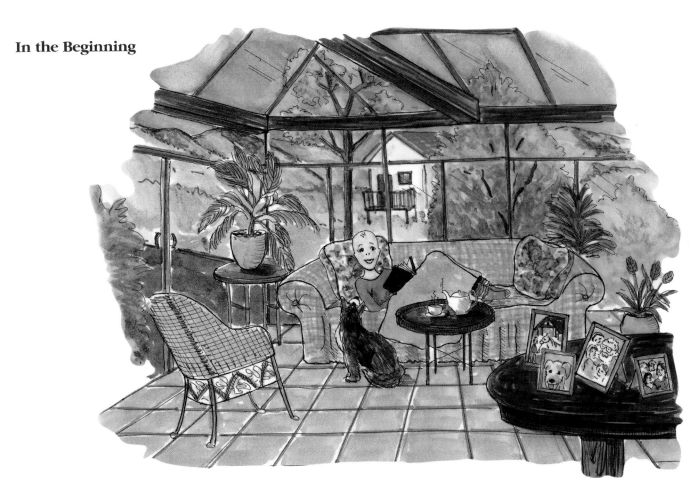

"Home Sweet Home" takes on a whole new meaning.

At Home

Where the heart is

Whether we are single, married, parents of small children or not, our homes take on a whole new light in the face of cancer. Unless we are very ill and need the medical security of a hospital, there is perhaps no other time when home becomes as crucial to our well-being.

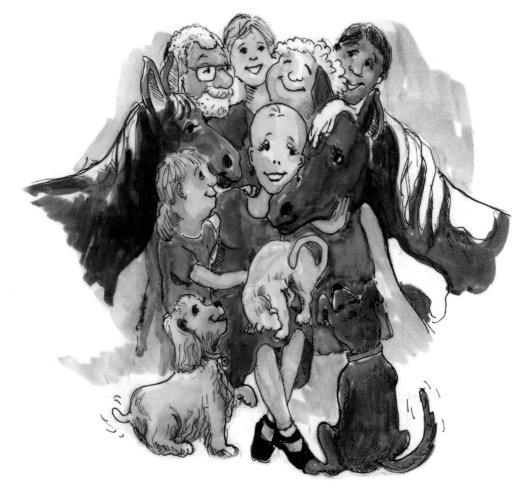

You will discover how loved you are.

It is here that we find warmth and familiarity after being so suddenly submerged in the icy, sterile waters of the cancer world. Home becomes our haven from the horridness of our disease.

Ironically, though, home can also be an ever-present reminder of all that we may lose. Cancer sheds painful, almost blinding light on the potential reality that we may have to say good-bye sooner than we wanted to those we love the most.

At Home

Something as simple as my little girl giving me a hug brought home to me that I may not be there to see her get married or even to help her as she crosses the threshold from girl to woman.

I found myself memorizing moments with my sons that I would normally take for granted. And as hard as I resisted doing so, I would envision and often resent another woman taking over my role as mother to them. How could anyone else love my kids as I do?

QUOTE

I am an old man and have known a great many troubles, but most of them have never happened.

—Mark Twain

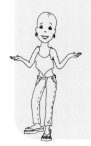

And what about my husband? As sweet and supportive as he was and still is, I find it difficult to accept the likelihood that he could spend his golden years with someone else.

But home is, indeed, where the heart is — and the heart is where joy and sorrow must live side by side. We all know we cannot have one without the other, but knowledge does not alleviate pain. Only faith, hope and love can soothe a life with seemingly more bitter than sweet.

At Home

Nevertheless, it is my hope that "home sweet home" will take

on a whole new meaning for you, as it did for me.

My home became a safe harbor for me to deal with the toxic

side effects of my chemotherapy regimen. I found comfort in

knowing that no matter how sick, scared or miserable my

treatments would render me, there would always be real rest,

love, and privacy for me at home.

HELPFUL HINTS

Take baths instead of showers…for relaxation and ease in keeping your catheter dry.

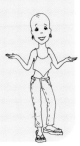

Ideally, our homes should be the one place where we can safely take off our scarves and wigs — and even our masks. Home should offer us the freedom to truly be ourselves in the midst of our new or not-so-new nightmare. It should be a refuge where we can safely vent our fears and tears.

At Home

Where the work is

Unfortunately, however, home is not only where the heart is but also where the work is — the housework! And if you're like me, the mess looks all the messier when the well-wishers bring in food or the looky-loos stop by for a visit.

With this in mind, it wasn't difficult to find the obvious advantages to being on chemotherapy at home. Of course, as with just about everything, it depends on one's perspective.

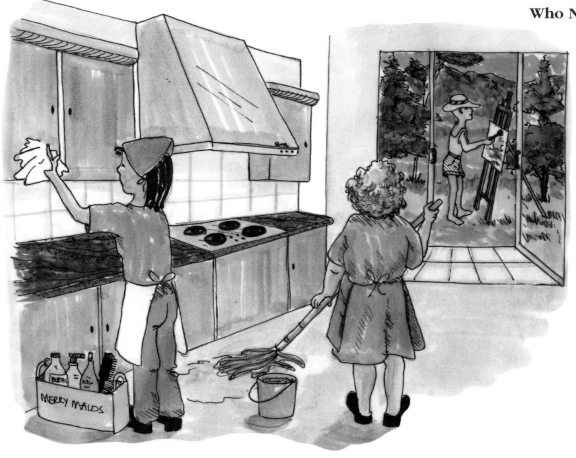

No more cleaning.

If you love to cook, then you'll have to take a break — or buy a new freezer for all the wonderful casseroles you'll probably receive. If you enjoy housework, well…you and I don't seem to have much in common, so I won't even go there. Nevertheless, if you are blessed, as I am, with lots of folks who want to help (and if you're not, then ask!), you will discover that your domestic duties have dwindled away to a bare minimum. This is temporary, so enjoy it.

HELPFUL HINTS

When friends ask what can they do for you, Ask them to….
- *bring you videos—only comedies and light hearted romances with happy endings!*
- *make you nurturing foods like tapioca, bread pudding and mild pasta dishes like Fettuccine Alfredo.*
- *bring you scarves or hats they aren't using*

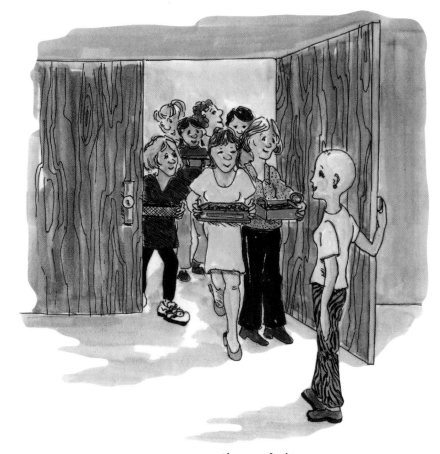

No more Cooking.

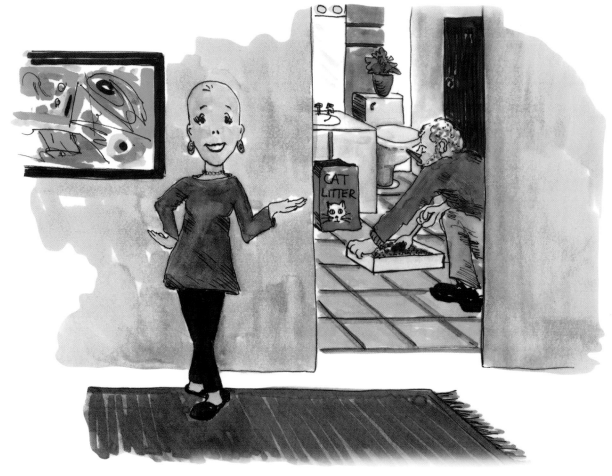

The Cat box is off limits—YES!

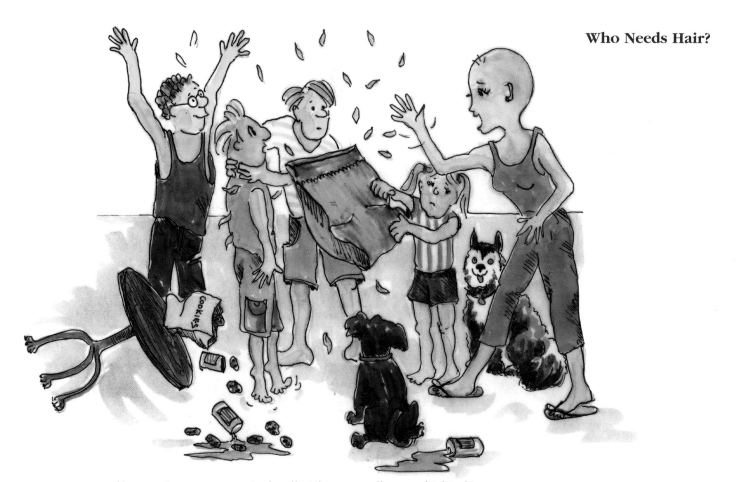

If you can't get your way, simply yell, "My cancer cells are multiplying!"

At Home

One wouldn't think that time flies during chemotherapy, but it does — especially in hindsight. Before I had a chance to get used to life *sans* housework, my eight-month chemotherapy regimen was completed, my hair was growing back and the dishes and laundry were mine to do again. The vast majority of us will have stable periods of remission, if not cure, during which our regular roles and routines return as quickly as they left us. So, again, take advantage of this time in your life to rest.

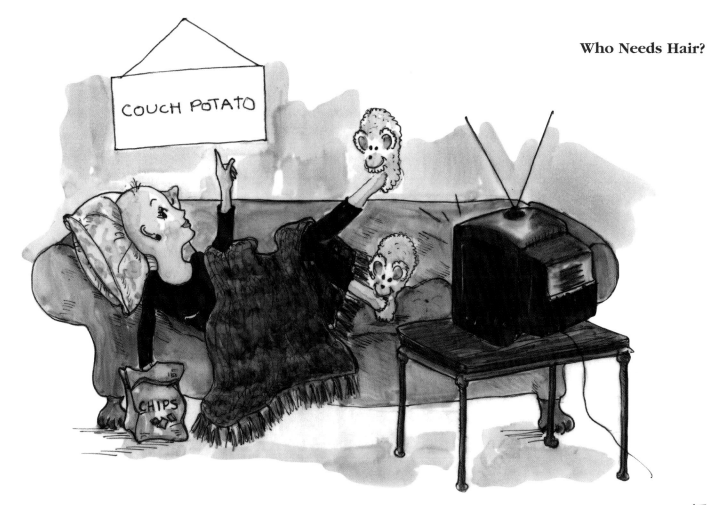

You now have a legitimate excuse to VEG.

Where we learn to "be"

Did I say rest? Yes, rest. Believe it or not, some people find this concept quite challenging. I did. I may hate housework, but sitting back and doing nothing was almost as equally uncomfortable for me. That is until I learned the art of "vegging" — you know, to make like a stalk of celery or something…just laying around and doing nada. This concept frightened me at first, for I equated vegging with being worthless

QUOTE

If you can spend a perfectly useless afternoon in a perfectly useless manner, you have learned to live.

—Lin Yutang

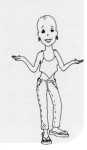

and, even worse, with inevitably rotting and smelling to the point of being thrown down the garbage disposal.

What I somehow missed along the way is that my self-worth comes not from what I do but from what I am. A person, a human being, a child of God. Yes, I know, most of us are happier when we are creative, productive and somewhat busy, but cancer taught me to just "be." To be still, to be aware, to live and love deliberately yet effortlessly...to be home.

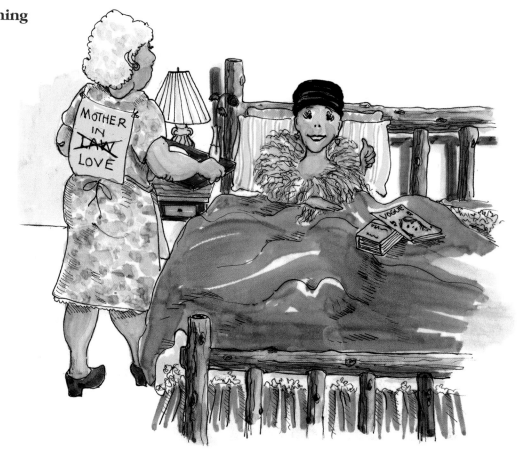

Your Mother-In-Law will like you!

HELPFUL HINTS

Order a TLC catalog for a great selection of hats, scarves, bangs and wigs. Call them at 1-800-227-2345 or online at www.cancer.org

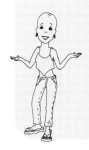

Out and About

Okay, ready, set, go…it's time to go out in public. My hair fell out sooner than I ever expected. I don't think even the video I saw at the hospital prepared me for the speed and utter completeness of my shedding. I remember thinking I might have a few weeks or so until all of my hair fell out. But as most of you know by now, it happens within days.

Out and About

Of course, my first instinct was to hide my hairless head at home. And who feels like going out anyway? But sooner or later, I realized that going on with my life meant going out in public and therefore was something with which I would have to get comfortable.

But, thankfully (I guess), the first few weeks of my indoctrination to cancer consisted mainly of staying home because I was so sick or tired that going out was unthinkable, unless it was

---

HELPFUL HINTS

For a brand new look...
Cute, Young Look:
Tie a bandana around your head and put on a baseball cap
Dramatic, Sexy, Gypsy Look:
Tie a scarf around your head (low on the forehead like a turbon) and then tie it over to the side
For the holidays or other special occasion:
Find a long sash or rectangular scarf in a festive color (maybe metallic gold) and tie around a basic black cotton cap.

HELPFUL HINTS

• ***Make Up Ideas:***
Try using a light brown eye pencil to draw in your eyebrows and line upper and lower eyelids. This will make a world of difference in easing your look as an obvious cancer patient.

And

• ***Don't forget earrings***
Choose classic gold or silver hoops, pearls, diamonds—to brighten your face, but stay away from tacky, flashy earrings for they will only do the opposite!

to the hospital or doctor for more treatments and tests.

I would put on a bandanna or scarf and a baseball cap and not worry too much about what I looked like. Not that you can't be cute in a bandanna and baseball cap! They just become old hat (pun intended) after a while, and you might want to do something a little different and perhaps dressier. After all, your hair does grow back sooner than you might think — but not that soon.

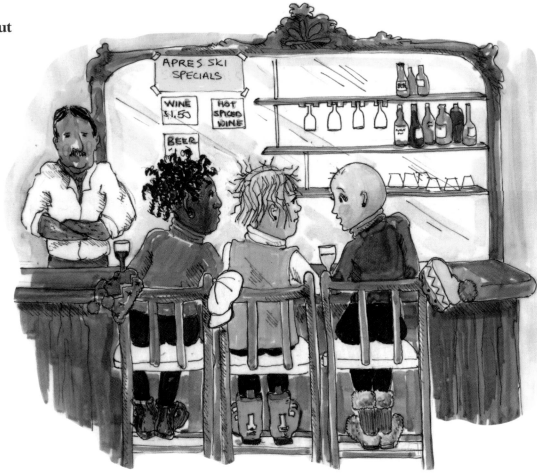

No more Hat Hair.

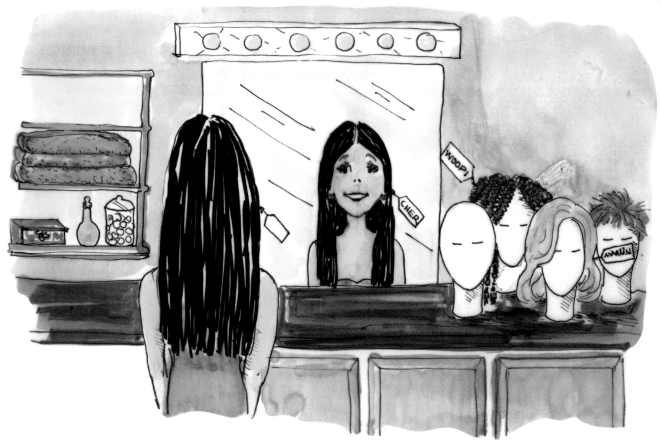

If wigs work for you...you can be a different women every day!

Out and About

Some of us will be confident or have a pretty-enough-shaped

head to just go bald. But if you have to go through chemother-

apy in the winter and you live anyplace that's the least bit

chilly, you will want to cover your head.

If you're lucky and really love your wig, then getting dressed

will be easy. But if you're like me, your wig(s) may not agree

with you. Not only did my head itch and sweat, but the mir-

ror reflected a strange and always crooked image back to me.

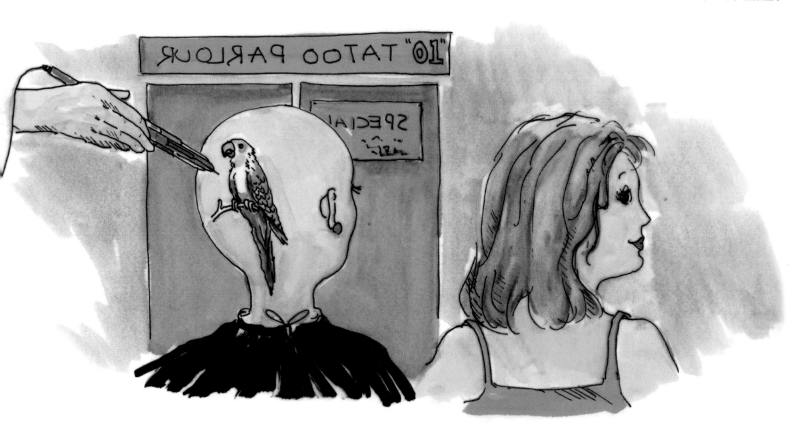

Now you can have that tatoo and not have to live with it forever.

55

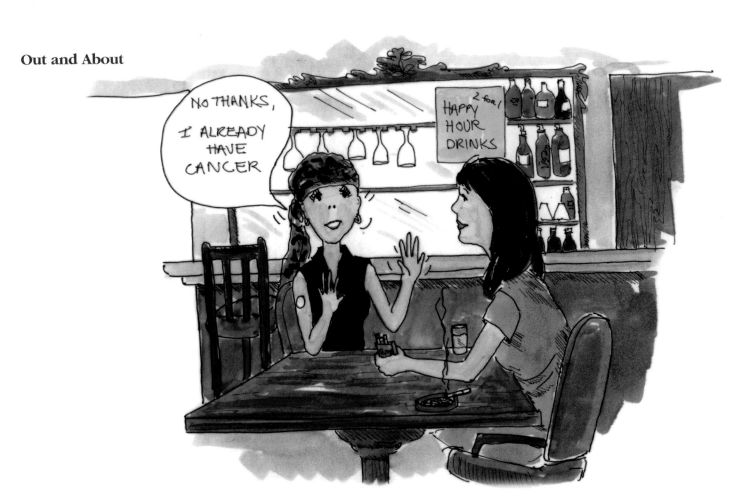

If you smoke, this will be your time to quit!

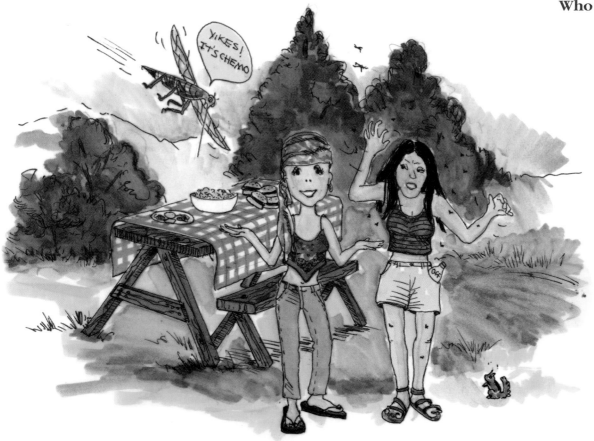

Mosquitoes won't like you anymore! really!

Out and About

Scarves became my cover-up of choice, and once I learned

how to tie them and adjust my wardrobe to match them, they

actually became kind of fun.

Learning how to "do" bald

My birthday came eight weeks after my diagnosis, and my

family wanted to take me out to dinner. It was my first real

night out since D-day (diagnosis day), and I remember feeling reasonably good and a bit excited about dressing up and going

out. I'll never forget going to my bedroom in hopes of finding

something pretty to wear. Instead, I came out in tears and

frustration.

Nothing in my beautiful new scarf collection matched any of

my old, not-so-beautiful clothes. All of my scarves were prints

and therefore clashed with the majority of my clothes —

which were also a variety of prints.

Out and About

Thus, I became enlightened. I needed a new wardrobe. My husband was thrilled when I announced this to him — bald, crying, on my birthday and in front of my parents. He said, "Sure, sweetheart, anything you need."

The good news for him, though, was that I didn't need a huge new wardrobe. Just a few new blouses and a couple of dresses in solid colors.

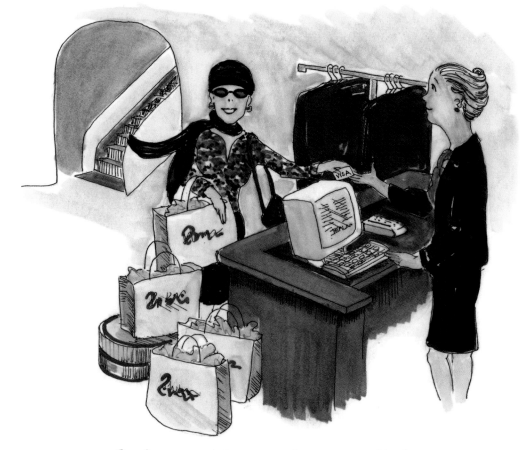

Time for a new wardrobe... to match your scarves and hats!

Once this seemingly simple realization sunk in to my newly

traumatized brain, getting dressed became a breeze. Almost as

easy as the drop of a hat! (I had to say it.) And my husband

was happier, too. Really.

In all honesty, whether the outing called for dressy or casual, I

could manage as long as I had a simple black dress, several

solid blouses — and lots of denim. I wore denim dresses,

HELPFUL HINTS

Basic Scarf Ideas:

- 3 or 4 cotton caps with and without side ties (preferably black and cream)
- 2 or 3 thick, braided headbands with Velcro closure to wrap around the above for going out.
- Find 3 or 4 printed scarves that you LOVE. (note: cotton ones will stay put best and feel most comfortable, but even with satin and silk ones, where there is a will, there is a way!)
- Use large square (fold over diagonally) and triangle scarves along with rectangular ones (at least, 12 inches wide)
- Fold down one edge about 3 or 4 inches and center this band against your forehead. Next, slide scarf to the right or left and tie over on side. If you have a large scarf you should be able to tuck the extra fold underneath the knot, giving you three swirls of material to adjust over one shoulder.

skirts, shirts and jeans, and they all blended nicely with just about any scarf.

I tried having some solid-colored scarves made but found that the prettier, jazzier ones covered a multitude of sins, including everything from the wrinkles in the fabric to the bumps on my head.

Silver or gold earrings went on next, along with a touch of eyeliner and eyebrow pencil to hide my lack of eyelashes and eyebrows.

I might have looked strange to others, but there were actually

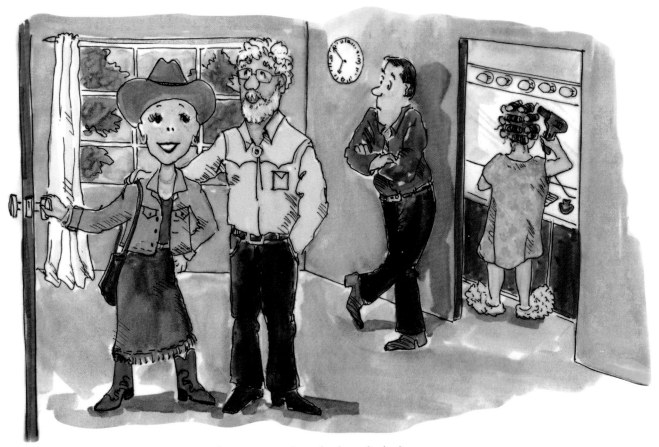

You can get ready at the drop of a hat!

HELPFUL HINTS

*Accomplish one thing
every day, no matter
how small.*

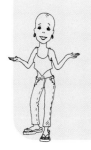

days when I liked my new look.

Whatever you may find easiest and/or more comfortable to do

with your new baldness — it is important to find something!

The American Cancer Society has a program called "Feel Good,

Look Good." And that says it all. We're not talking vanity here.

We're talking about going on with our lives in lieu of shutting

ourselves up in our homes until our nightmare is over and our

hair grows back.

The point is, we may discover that our nightmare is a lot more

Out and About

tolerable once we wake up and become active again. First,

maybe a walk. Next, perhaps the grocery store, and then,

maybe lunch with a friend.

But beware. It's a curious world that awaits to check us out.

Some people have a morbid curiosity to see the effects of such

a dramatic thing as chemo—you know, the so-called "looky-loos."

HELPFUL HINTS

Take a walk everyday you can!…
for your muscles, joints, moods and more.

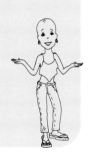

And, of course, just plain good folks will need to see that we are doing okay.

Helping others "do" bald

Actually, I think our going out in public helps to break the ice for others. I learned from my experience that others were more frightened than I about encountering me back in the "real" world. Once the initial greeting and/or hug and/or acknowledgment was over with, so was the awkwardness.

Out and About

On a larger scale, our helping others become more

comfortable with our predicament can have far greater

ramifications than we may know. Cancer can be a lonely

place, even for the most loved and adored of us.

I have felt this loneliness…in a crowded restaurant, in a movie

theater, at a dinner party with friends, even sitting amongst

my beautiful family. I simply have felt *alone*, as if no one

around me truly knew my plight.

I've often played a little mental game with myself in a crowded place such as a shopping mall or airport. I imagine myself yelling out, "Hey! Who here has cancer? Raise your hand!" And then maybe four or five people slowly stop talking or walking and look at me and raise their hands. We simply smile warmly at one another as if to say, "We're okay. We're not alone. We can do this." And then everyone goes on about their business and I imagine we're all just a little bit stronger.

Out and About

I cannot fathom how lonely cancer must have been for all the brave people who pioneered this epidemic. But brave people they were and the surviving ones still are. Unfortunately, now it is our turn to pave the way for others and, hopefully, this sense of isolation will ease and lessen with time.

So venture out and about. Your public presence will not only make others more comfortable but will make you feel better in a multitude of little ways.

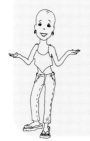

HELPFUL HINTS

Go outside each day if you can for fresh air and a LITTLE bit of sunshine.
Remember, though--some chemotherapy can make you ultra sensitive to the sun.

That is IF you are feeling up to it and your blood cell count is normal so as not to put you at risk.

Which brings us to the next chapter.

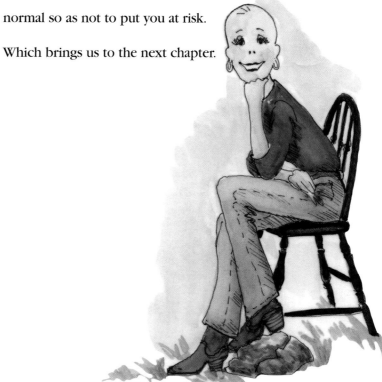

71

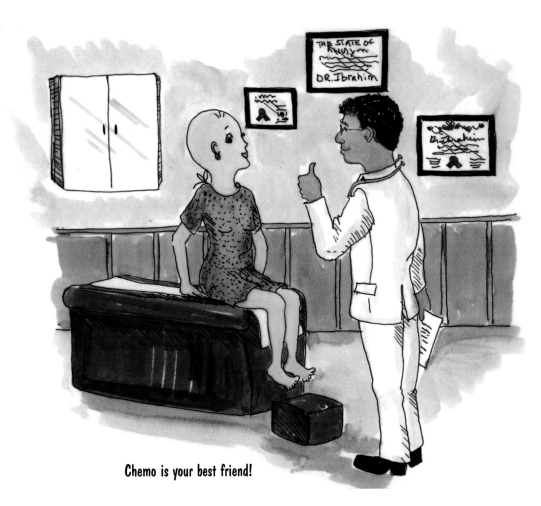

Chemo is your best friend!

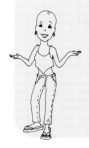
Physically and Personally

There is probably no harsher medical treatment than chemotherapy. Poisonous to our healthy cells as well as our cancerous ones, the grueling effect of chemotherapy on the body is notorious. In fact, before cancer threatened my life, I was one of those uninformed and just plain scared folks who said, "If I ever get cancer, I'll never subject my body to chemotherapy." I used to think that almost any alternative was safer and perhaps wiser than chemotherapy. But when the Big C becomes *your* diagnosis, and doctors who have devoted their lives to oncology recommend this course of treatment, you will, hopefully, do your research and find that in the majority of cases chemotherapy may be your greatest ally. I am not discounting the possibility of other treatments being helpful, but more and more people are being cured, or their cancer is being treated and *controlled*, as a result of chemotherapy.

HELPFUL HINTS

Do NOT take mega-doses of any vitamin or food supplement without the knowledge of your doctor.

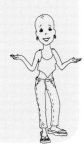

HELPFUL HINTS

Be patient with yourself during chemotherapy. Find your cycle of down days and up days so you can plan accordingly.

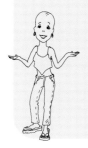

Even the harsh side effects are diminishing somewhat through the use of other medicines given before, during and after chemo. But diminishing or not, these side effects are still hefty challenges for even the strongest of us to endure. Most chemotherapy agents deplete the white blood cell count, which severely compromises the immune system, rendering us susceptible to other illnesses. The red blood cell count also drops drastically, which gives new meaning to the concept of "fatigue."

Physically and Personally

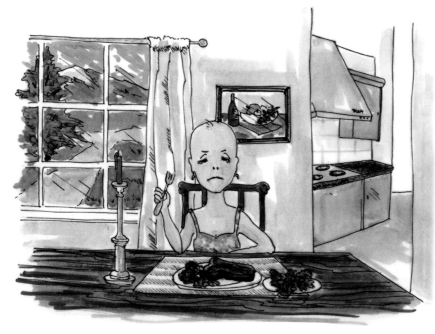

You are now eligible for Trauma Trim.

We can suffer extreme nausea, vomiting and diarrhea. Our mouths may become full of ulcers and sores so painful that even drinking a milk shake through a straw is unbearable. Our feet and hands can tingle so painfully due to nerve damage that only submerging them in bowls of ice water will help.

These are just some of the harsh physical realities of chemotherapy. Fortunately, things have come a long way in terms of reducing the miserable side effects of this treatment.

HELPFUL HINTS

Prevent mouth sores by using baking soda & peroxide toothpaste (only) and gargling daily with salt & baking soda mix.

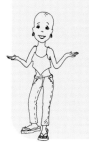

With a primary diagnosis being of Stage Four advanced breast cancer, my best option appeared to be a trial study which involved a chemotherapy cocktail of Adriamycin and Taxol. All of the above-mentioned side effects became a part of my life for many months. Yet with every checkup, I became closer and closer to partial and then complete remission.

Yes, my cancer had spread to my bones, which is (at present) an incurable condition, but my chemotherapy regimen took control and, thankfully, put my cancer into what my daughter

Physically and Personally

calls "hibernation." "Mama," she still says to this day, when the

flip side, along with faith, seem to elude even me, "remember,

just like with the bears, your cancer has gone into a long,

long hibernation."

So this is the paradox of chemotherapy. What makes you sick

can make you well. This mixed bag of blessings called

chemotherapy destroys the healthy as well as the unhealthy

cells within our bodies. The good news is that our healthy

cells rebuild themselves quicker than the cancer cells, so with

QUOTE

I have learned never to underestimate the capacity of the human mind and body to regenerate— even when the prospects seem most wretched.

—Norman Cousins,
Anatomy of an Illness

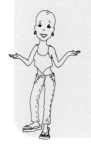

the deliberate and strategic application of chemotherapy agents, we have a good shot at staying ahead of the game. Yes, we pay the price in the short term for what we hope has long-term results. Fortunately, our miraculous bodies hold a life force and a natural healing system that can bounce back from even the assault of chemotherapy. As Louise L. Hay put it, "Be assured that every day, your body's natural desire is to be healthy, whole, and complete." This revelation gave me a new sense of admiration for a body I had previously taken for

Physically and Personally

granted during much of my life. And then, strangely, it was time to go to war.

Another paradox or incongruity in the world of cancer arises when we begin to perceive a battle being fought within our own bodies — just as we are learning to love and appreciate them as perhaps never before. War lingo is used to describe all aspects of the cancer patient's ordeal. In life, we are portrayed as brave soldiers who are mighty warriors against a hideous disease. Yet in death, many of our eulogizers speak of us as losing or succumbing to our battle with cancer.

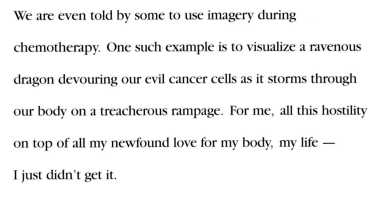

QUOTE

Above all else, for optimum health and healing, love yourself more and more each day!

—Louise L. Hay

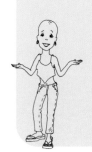

We are even told by some to use imagery during chemotherapy. One such example is to visualize a ravenous dragon devouring our evil cancer cells as it storms through our body on a treacherous rampage. For me, all this hostility on top of all my newfound love for my body, my life — I just didn't get it.

A friend called me one day not long after my diagnosis.

Physically and Personally

We talked about the "battle" I was facing, and he offered advice I very much needed to hear. He said to get rid of the hostility and begin to think lovingly about all of my cells — even the imbalanced, malignant, so-called "bad" ones. He taught me to view the whole process of getting well with love, patience and admiration.

Suddenly, I was talking to my cancer cells as if they were merely wayward children who needed to get hold of themselves. It may sound crazy, but the loss of hostility immediately felt wonderful, and my new patience and love for even my wayward, out-of-balance cells felt somehow good, right and necessary. For I soon discovered that my abnormal, malignant cells were as much a part of my body as my other cells, and we were all in this together. We needed camaraderie, not hostility.

You may prefer the active combat mode for your own personal strategy against cancer. Whatever works or whatever feels right to you will usually be the right course. And this doesn't mean we can't drift in and out of different modes as we learn to cope with the uncertainties and unpredictability of cancer.

Physically and Personally

I fully realize that if and when my disease progresses, I may engage in an all-out battle of my own, with no arms barred. I suppose we cancer patients do fight a private war within ourselves, whether we realize it or not. We must struggle almost continually to cope with not only the harsh effects of treatment but also with our new very unwanted status as a cancer patient.

As we work through these struggles, learning to balance strength with surrender will be one of the most important things we can do for ourselves.

QUOTE

Remember that nature is a great healer.
Even small doses will begin to restore your sense of balance, joy, and wonder.
When you return to your source, your soul is fed.

—Louise L Hay

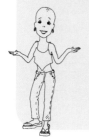

When do we push ourselves and when do we just let go and succumb to what our bodies are telling us? Another friend, Annie Pringle, a neuromuscular massage therapist, taught me the importance of learning when to let go and when to hold on. There are simply those times when surrender is all we can do. But to do it and do it fully, without guilt, is sometimes trickier than one may think, especially for those of us who are accustomed to being busy and productive.

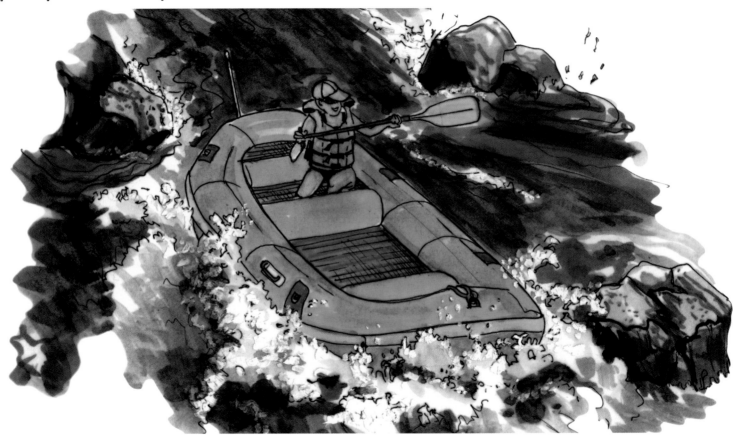

You will learn the art of Holding on & Letting Go!

HELPFUL HINTS

Each day, get up, get dressed, and put on a little make-up. Pretend someone unexpected is coming—it will brighten your mood.....
even if you go right back to bed.

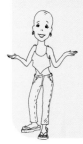

By the same token, forcing ourselves to get up and take that walk can demand more energy than we cancer patients can muster. But when our muscles and joints become painful from lack of use and our souls become weary, a little strength goes a long way.

Physically and Personally

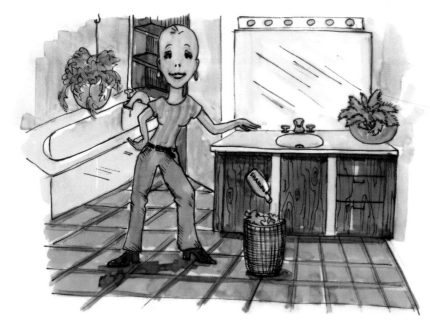

No Need to buy shampoo, conditioner, mouse, gel, hairspray, etc!

On a lighter note, there is something to be said for not having to shave your legs or pluck your eyebrows anymore. I did have to learn how to draw eyebrows, and if I had to pick, I would certainly pick plucking over drawing, but hey, I enjoyed the break.

How about you? Can you possibly find any joy (however itty-bitty) in not having to buy shampoo or get your hair highlighted? It may take practice, but I read somewhere that attitude is the mind's paintbrush. It can color any situation.

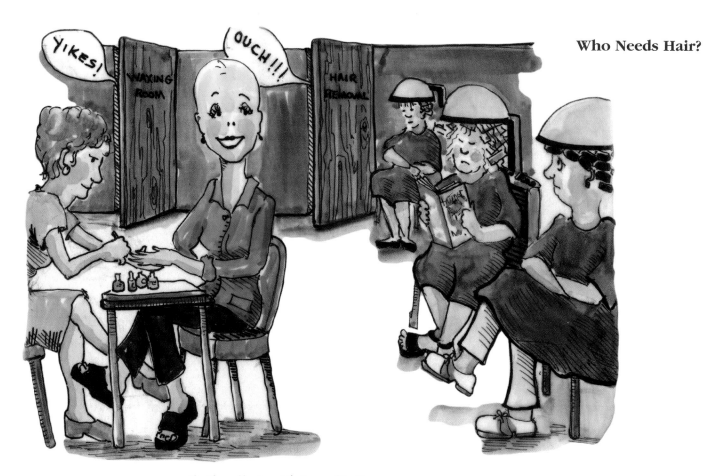

No More Shaving, Waxing or Plucking

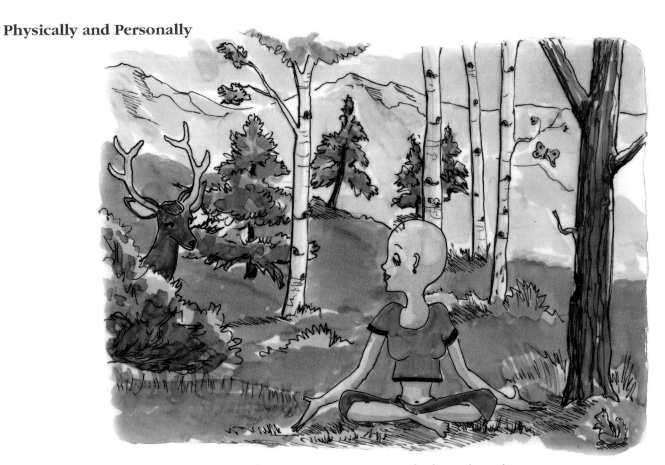

This is your greatest opportunity for Spiritual growth.

QUOTE

God is teaching me through all this to rediscover the substance of my strength and song. Perhaps this is an unusual opportunity to discover who I really am….

—Tim Hansel, *You Gotta Keep Dancin'*

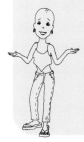

Spiritually

The whole cancer experience is so bizarre and surreal that it would seem impossible not to reflect on one's spiritual side. Suddenly catapulted into a frightening and foreign land, we are forced to question everything we've ever known to be true, or at least normal.

Spiritually

Our hair falls out, some of us lose our breasts to surgery, our bodies are deliberately poisoned, or so it would seem — and perhaps most challenging is coming face to face with our own mortality.

If the above still renders you numb to the status of your spiritual dimension, then how about the following? What is the first thing every card, flower, phone call, e-mail and visitor says to you upon your diagnosis? You got it! "I'm praying for you."

Of course, the new-agers say they're sending us light and lighting candles and incense for us. Some Native and not-so-Native

QUOTE

Feed your faith and doubt will starve to death

—anonymous

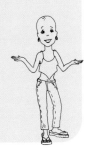

American friends even gave me medicine bags that contained healing stones to rub.

Everyone meant well, and being the spiritually receptive person I am — not to mention a bit desperate due to my situation, I embraced everyone's attempt to save me from death and/or eternal damnation. How else do you respond to a person offering prayer? "Oh, please don't. It might interfere with my chemotherapy." Ha! Even the most self-proclaimed atheist would be hard pressed to respond with that.

Spiritually

But for me, this insidious disease which threatened my physical life became the very medicine that enriched my spirituality.
When I was about four weeks into chemo, bald as an eagle,
nauseous, exhausted and numb with fear and shock, I had a
very real (to me) supernatural experience.

I was putting my little girl, Alden, barely eight years old, to
sleep. Thankfully, the chaos of cancer had at least left her
bedtime ritual untouched. Mommy may be bald, and mommy
may be sick, but mommy could still sing, read, hug and love.

And sing I did on this particular night. A bit out of tune, as usual, but nevertheless I sang. With my bare head settled on her pillow and my precious child snuggled up against my shoulder, I sang every word of every song (may I brag?) in my four-song repertoire — which includes (why stop now?) "Somewhere Over the Rainbow," "Summertime," "Hush Little Baby" and "Amazing Grace." I've always sung these songs to my kids at bedtime, at least until they got tired of my voice or until the ritual slowly faded away like childhood itself. But, on the night of my experience, after somehow getting through each song, I laid there mesmerized by how beautiful

Spiritually

my sleeping child looked slumped down on my chest, eyes
closed, mouth slightly open and full cheeks relaxed. And then
the thoughts.

*Oh…would I be there to see her face change ever so slowly
and gracefully from child to woman? Or would I only know
her face as a child?* And, more painful. *Would she remember
my face, my songs, my love?* I tried to blink back tears and
remembered my eyelashes were gone. *Oh, what a mess. Oh,
what a nightmare.*

I managed to untangle myself from my daughter without waking her, and then I did what I always do over each of my children's sleeping bodies before I leave their rooms at night. I cross them. By that I mean I take my thumb and sketch an imaginary cross over their bodies. It's just a little protection thing I do, a way of wordless prayer, of lifting my babies up before I leave them for the night.

As I turned to leave after crossing my daughter, I suddenly sensed a strong yet gentle force lift my own hand to my forehead, then down over my stomach and then up from one

Spiritually

shoulder to the other. Stunned, I realized I had just sketched

an invisible cross over myself— something I have rarely done

except shyly a few times at the communion rail of my hus-

band's Episcopal church.

Amazed, and a little shaken, I turned to my child's window,

and as I looked out at a sky overflowing with stars, it dawned

on me that I had forgotten something very important. All

these wonderful people were praying for me and I had not

even thought to pray for myself.

You see, in recent years, I had become very lax, or should I say "vague," about my spirituality. This would not be strange except that for most of my life I had been a deeply religious Christian. For many reasons, most having to do with pride, I had let go of traditional religion, which in and of itself would have been fine — if I had not also let go of my relationship with God.

In my desire to be open to all paths of spirituality, I had unknowingly stepped off my own path, which led to lethargy and a certain laziness. I didn't know that "use it or lose it" applies to our faith as well as our IQ.

Spirituality

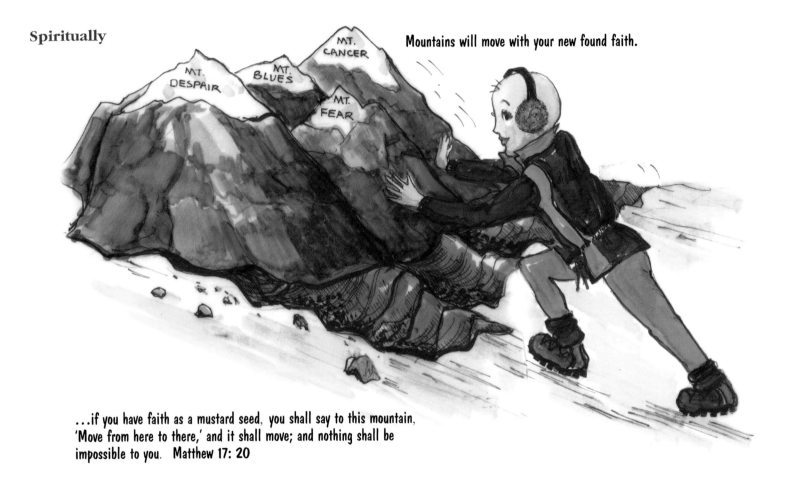

Mountains will move with your new found faith.

...if you have faith as a mustard seed, you shall say to this mountain, 'Move from here to there,' and it shall move; and nothing shall be impossible to you.   Matthew 17: 20

Cancer showed me that illness can indeed be a reset button

for all areas our lives — especially our spirituality. Perhaps Dr.

Larry Dossey, in *Meaning and Medicine,* says it best when he

quotes one of his colleagues, Brad Lemley: "We tend to think

that the purpose of prayer is to terminate sickness, but we for-

get that the purpose of sickness may be to initiate prayer, or,

more generally, a consciousness of the Infinite."

For me, this meant acknowledging a power greater than

myself — even greater than my *higher self.* In my life before

cancer, I had so successfully navigated the course of my own and even my family's lives — or so I thought — that I had

begun to believe I could control just about anything.

Not true with cancer. Some will say, "But Sallie, you

controlled your cancer with your positive thinking." Not so. I

controlled my *attitude* by choosing joy instead of misery, but

cancer was a different animal for even *me*, "Miss Sunshine," to

tame.

This was why relief, as well as awe, encompassed me on that

special evening in my daughter's room. I didn't have to be in

charge anymore.

QUOTE

Whatever is true, whatever is honorable, whatever is right, whatever is pure, whatever is lovely, whatever is of good repute, if there is any excellence and if anything worthy of praise, let your mind dwell on these things.

—Philippians 4:8

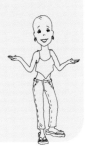

Some will think you're special.

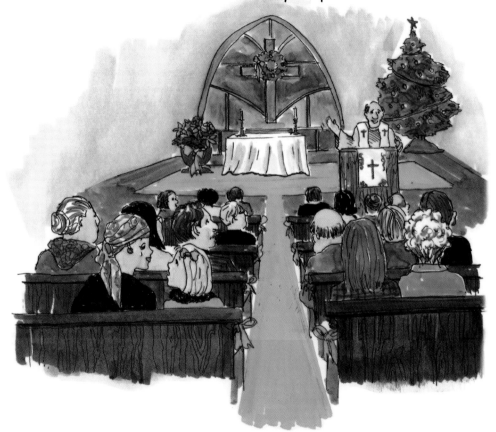

"Mama, you're special. You're the only one here on Chemo"

Spiritually

Whether an angel or a narcotic-induced me or God *Himself* lifted my hand that night did not matter. What did matter was that a tiny seed of faith began to stir anew within my soul. Suddenly I knew that the overall outcome of my health was — and would continue to be — in hands much bigger than my own. In hands even bigger than my brilliant and beloved doctors'.

Simultaneously, as my faith in a real and loving Creator increased, the burden to be the perfect cancer patient decreased. Yes, I wanted to educate and take care of myself, yet the overwhelming responsibility had lifted.

QUOTE

I will lead the blind by ways they have not known, along unfamiliar paths. I will guide them, I will turn the darkness into light before them and make the rough places smooth. These are the things I will do; I will not forsake them.

—Isaiah 42:16

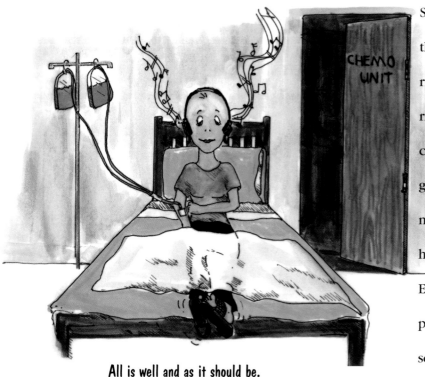

All is well and as it should be.

So often, we cancer patients are pressured to think the right thoughts, to use imagery the right way, to eat the right foods, to take the right vitamins and supplements, etc. Why, one could get cancer again just from the stress of getting over the first bout. The point is, we need to relax and not crucify ourselves if we have a few bad moments or some junk food. Even so, I did find it helpful to have a phrase or prayer to meditate upon when I was especially scared or feeling pessimistic.

Spiritually

I would say, "All is well and as it should be" over and over until it became *real* to me. This phrase securely anchored me many times during the toughest times of my treatments. Just the mere utterance of these words filled my heart with peace. In essence, my phrase was simply a declaration to myself of a bigger picture in the madness I was facing.

A young woman named Shannon, whom I have gotten to know at a local cancer center, has taught me much about this faith of which I speak. She is a leukemia patient in her twenties, yet she is wiser than most women four times her age. Shannon told me that cancer's greatest gift to her was the lesson of humility.

> ## QUOTE
>
> *Slowly my rage to live emerged from the depression, frustration, and anger. But when it was there I realized that it had a task to it that I'd never known before. I began to see life in a way that never would have been possible before. I began to relish small, daily, simple things—and realized at a depth that never seemed possible that ALL of life was sacred. There were moments, though sporadic and far apart, when I began to understand that life wasn't over for me— but perhaps just beginning.*
>
> —Tim Hansel, You Gotta Keep Dancin'

Ha, you say — some gift. Yet to her, and to me, this humility she speaks of is not for wimps and willy-nillys, but for the strongest of souls. As you well know by now, it is no easy task to do all you can humanly do and then sit back and TRUST. Yes, TRUST. In your doctor, in your treatments, in your body's natural life force, in a loving God who created you and cares for you. That is humility. To know that whether or not we survive this disease is not up to us. And above all, to know that no matter what, all is well and as it should be. **And when it's all said and done, who needs hair anyway?**

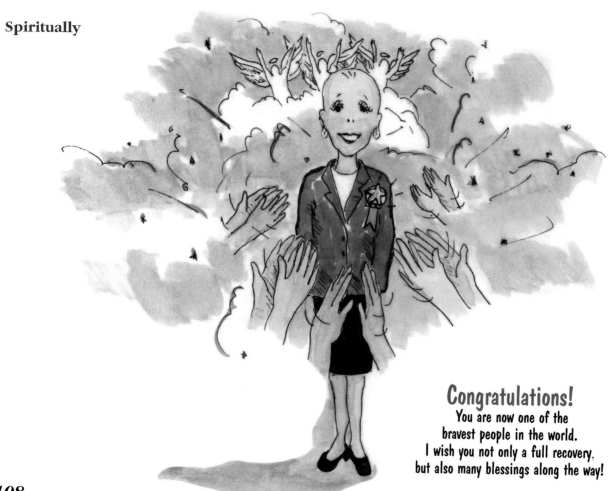

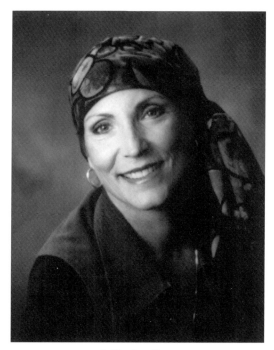

Sallie Burdine

About the Author

Sallie Burdine was diagnosed with Stage Four advanced breast cancer in July of 1998. She had just begun her career as a writer when cancer invaded her life. On the day of her diagnosis, she mailed her finished manuscript entitled Midlife Women UNPLUGGED…at last! to her agent in New York. As Sallie underwent chemotherapy for her metastasized breast cancer, she sought daily to find the blessings in her curse, which became the catalyst for Who Needs Hair.

Sallie's mother and sister are also breast cancer survivors. Sallie lives with her husband, Hank, and their three children, Matt, Ben and Alden, in Bluewater Bay, Florida and is presently at work on *The Surprising Blessings in Cancer.*

About the Illustrator

In addition to being a fine artist, Becky Kieler is a co-warrior in the fight against cancer. After both of her parents became victims of cancer, Becky joined the Colorado Marrow Donor Program in 1992. A year later, she was a "miracle match" to a 9-month-old little girl with leukemia. Becky donated her marrow and gave the gift of life to "Jasmine," who is now seven years old.

Becky's impressionistic landscapes have been displayed at art shows and galleries throughout Colorado. Her background also includes seventeen years as an ABC Television courtroom artist. Her illustrations have been published in numerous articles and periodicals. She is also involved in mural painting and graphic design for homes and businesses in the Denver area. Becky lives with her husband, Michael, and their dog, Winston, in Genessee, Colorado.

www.brushinhand.com

becky@brushinhand.com

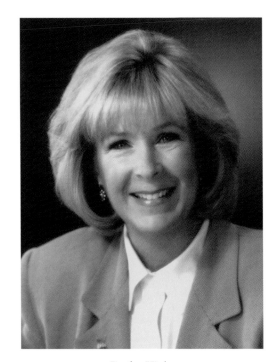

Becky Kieler

Highlights to Remember

- *Choose each morning to live life fully with joy and thanksgiving while remembering that NOBODY is promised a tomorrow.*

- *Strive to get up and get dressed, even if you go back to bed.*

- *Put on a smile, even if it feels false…at first.*

- *Spend your day as your energy dictates with peace and patience for what your body is going through.*

- *Move your body every day -- whether you simply stretch or take a walk.*

- *Breathe deeply and purposefully and go outside for fresh air.*

- *Drink sufficient water.*

- *Accomplish one thing every day — no matter how small.*

CUT ALONG DOTTED LINE

Quick Order Form

FAX ORDERS: 850-897-8271. Send this form.
TELEPHONE ORDERS: Call 866-897-SABA toll free, (273-7222)Have your credit card ready.
E-MAIL ORDERS: sababooks@aol.com
POSTAL ORDERS: SABA Books, P.O. Box 5265, Bluewater Bay, FL 32578

Please send the following Books. I understand that I may return any of them for a full refund—for any reason, no questions asked.

_____

_____

NAME _____

ADDRESS_____

CITY_____**STATE** _____

ZIP _____

TELEPHONE_____

E-MAIL _____

PAYMENT:
☐ **CHECK**   ☐ **CREDIT CARD**
☐ Visa   ☐ MasterCard   ☐ AMEX   ☐ Discover

CARD#: _____

NAME ON CARD: _____

EXP.DATE _____

Sales tax: Please add 6% for products shipped to Florida address.

Shipping: US: $4.00 for the first book and $2.00 for each additional product.

_____
SIGNATURE HERE

SABA
B O O K S
Post Office Box 5265
Bluewater Bay, Florida 32578
TOLL FREE 866-273-7222

Highlights to Remember (continued)

- *Remember to add humor to your life — which has been proven to boost our immune systems, reduce our stress levels, and add life to our days, if not days to our lives!*

- *Protect your privacy and time without guilt. Be a little selfish.*

- *Nurture an attitude of gratitude by writing down 3-5 things you are thankful for each night before going to sleep.*

But, still…

- *Allow yourself to have periods of anger, fear and sadness. Acknowledging and accepting these feelings are prerequisites for finding the Flip side!*

And above all…

*Feed your faith and recognize the Creator of your body and soul.
"Draw near to God, and He will draw near to you."*

—James 4:8